Midnight:
Anti-Trafficking
Medical Anthology

To our patients, & human trafficking victims & survivors; to anti-trafficking allies & advocates, & those who protect our daughters, sons, brothers, sisters, mothers, fathers, cousins, nephews, & nieces & all whom we love

PREFACE

We all want to be free. None of us deserves to be enslaved. Not women, not men, not girls, and not boys. No one deserves to be kidnapped and abused, misled, or misused. Hear the representative strong voice of victims and survivors of human trafficking, specifically sex trafficking, within the pages of these poems and on the cover of this book.

Share these widely to spread awareness and build a better future – for all.

Sherry-Ann Brown, MD, PhD
@drbrowncares
drbrowncares@gmail.com
www.drbrowncares.com

TABLE OF CONTENTS

PART ONE

Prologue

If You Knew,
Would you
Do something?

If you were moved
By these words
About victims
In your backyard
Or on your front porch,
Would you
Do something?

PART TWO

Sacred Spaces

As I sat at dinner,
Eating lobster,
Cracked open
By a colleague
Next to me,
And torn apart
By the waiter
Gently and kindly,
I looked outside
The open doors
To Bourbon Street,
In New Orleans,
After a long day
Of great discussions
At a national medical conference.

Across the street,
I saw a girl
Scantily clad
And leaning against
The door jam,
And I saw a guy approach her.

I sighed,
Lowered my eyes,
To the lobster,
And turned
And looked at my colleague.
I said,
"It hurts
My heart

To know
That
There is quite likely
Human trafficking occurring
Right across the street
Before our eyes."

He
Made a thought-provoking
Comment
About prostitution
And human trafficking.

After dinner,
I walked along Bourbon Street
Headed back to my hotel,
Hanging onto the arm
Of a colleague.

Something spilled,
And I needed
A tissue
Or a napkin
Or something
To mop it up.
To cover it over.
As if it wasn't there.

A lady
Standing outside of
An establishment
On Bourbon Street
Said to me,
"Wait! I'll get you something.

Let me help you."
I smiled at her kindness,
And said, "Thank you!"
She returned immediately
With a clean napkin.
As I wiped up the mess,
I looked up at the establishment.
Behind her was a door jam.
Through it, on the wall,
Were pictures
That were
Too X-rated
For my eyes.
Even my patients wear gowns.
Well, most of them.
Some try not to.
My colleague made a comment
About where the napkin
Might have come from.
He wondered
Whether
A woman
May have been violated
At some point in time
To afford us this napkin.
After using the napkin
To wipe up my mess,
I felt violated,
On some woman's behalf.
That was on Bourbon Street
In New Orleans.

Do you know
That the Super Bowl in New Orleans

Was reportedly home
To one of
The biggest human trafficking events
In 2016?
Every year actually,
The Super Bowl
Is one of
The largest human trafficking events
In the United States.
Yes,
In the United States;
Not only in Nicaragua,
Nepal,
Or any of those other places
You might think of.

OK,
So maybe
You don't watch
The Super Bowl.

Maybe
You
Don't watch football at all.
Maybe you didn't see
The game
In which
The Broncos
Beat
The New Orleans Saints.
The Saints.
In 2016.
The day before
I found myself sitting

In a restaurant
With my colleague
Cracking open
Lobster,
And the waiter
Tearing apart
The meaty flesh
Of the lobster,
Gently
And kindly,
On Bourbon Street,
Right across from
A young girl
Scantily clad
And leaning
Against
The door jam,
While a man
Approached her.
Maybe you didn't see that game.

Maybe
You
Didn't see
The emails,
Brochures,
Flyers,
Newsletters,
Bulletins,
Or news items
From local, regional, national,
And international organizations
Committed
To protecting

Her sacred spaces.

That victims and survivors know
What some were looking at last night.
On the computer.
Alone.
That anti-trafficking advocates know
That girls and boys
And men and women
In your hometown and state
Are being used
And abused
And mistreated,
And that their spaces
Are not being considered sacred.
Maybe you didn't see
The opportunities for you
To serve alongside
Your local or regional organizations,
And county attorneys,
Victims,
Survivors,
Allies,
Advocates,
And sergeants
To protect
Our daughters and
Our sons,
Our brothers
And our sisters,
Our mothers
And our fathers,
Our cousins
And our nephews,

Our nieces
And our grandkids,
Right in our own backyards
And on our front porches.

It is not only in New Orleans
And on Bourbon Street.
It is not only in the French Quarter.
It is not only during the Super Bowl.
It is not only in Nicaragua,
Nepal,
Or any of those other places
You might think of.
Sex trafficking is pervasive
Across the United States of America.

On the cold winter nights,
When you and I might be cozy
At home in our warm blankets
By the fire,
Turning the pages
Of a good book,
Or The Good Book,
Or looking at the front page
Of this week's newspaper,
There are many looking at Backpage.
More than willing to meet
In the icy bitter cold.
And violate
Sacred spaces.

PART THREE

Live Another Day

Why doesn't she just leave?
Why does she respond to the man
Walking up to her
While she is scantily clad
And leaning
Against the door jamb?

Perhaps if she could
Write a haiku, she might say,
"Live another day."

She might tell you how
Exploitation really works --
How she has no voice;

She might tell you that
He still controls her with crack,
And hides money 'round back.

She might tell you, since
He knows her mother's address,
She puts on this dress.

PART FOUR

Reach For The Stars

Did you know
That X-rated stars,
When they were growing up,
Did not think
That was what it meant
When their mothers said,
"Reach for the stars"?
Did you know
That while they are growing up,
Many are kidnapped
And bred
And fed
To be trafficked?

If you knew,
What would you do?
Would you do something?

Would you help
Spread the word
About informative events?
Would you find
Ways to help
Locally
Wherever
You
Find yourself?
Would you serve
As an advocate?
An ally?

Would you help
Give victims
A choice?
Would you help
Give survivors
A voice?
Would you help us
Find a way
To reacclimatize
The survivor,
Reintegrate
The victim,
And rehabilitate
The oppressor?

Would you help us
Educate johns?
Would you help
Bring backpage
To the front page?

Or would you
Simply
Turn the page?

How much
Of your empathy
Do you think
It's worth
To help
Each victim
See her worth?

How much
Of your time
Realistically
Would you want
To spare
To give
A survivor dignity?

How much
Of your power
Would you use
To save a child
From being trafficked
Another hour?

Do you know
The signs?
Do you know
The questions?
Do you know
What to do?
What would
You do?
Would you
Do something?

Would you
Spread awareness or
Lend a hand?

Would you
Change policy,
Work for

Social justice,
Or fight
For human rights?

Would you
Fight
For the human voice,
And for worth
And dignity?

Would you
Use your power
So that she
Doesn't have to stand
Scantily clad
In the doorjamb
Another hour?

Speaking of power...

PART FIVE

A Digital Exposé

Computer failures
Were predicted for Y2K.

Moral failures
As well,
Except
Moral failures
Have no timeline.
Yet, his came
In Y2K as well.

On his computer.
In the year 2000.

Popped up.
Shocked.
Curious.
Interested.
Fascinated.

When he looked,
He didn't know.

When he stared,
He didn't know.

What if he knew?
Would those moments
Have been different?

He explored his young naïveté

Every once in a while
Over a few months.

Then God's Spirit arrested him
In his tracks.

He didn't know.
What if he knew?
Would it have made a difference?

Had he known
That each image
Was made popular
By each woman's
Self-esteem
Being
Cut
At the jugular,
I wish
It would have
Made a difference.

I wish that instead
It would have gone:

Popped up.
Shocked.
NOT Curious.
NOT Interested.
NOT Fascinated.
Horrified.
Broken inside.
For those women.
Their bodies objectified.

When he looked,
He didn't know.

When he stared,
He didn't know.

What if he knew?
Would those moments
Have been different?

They should
Have been different.

Because God was watching,
And because they were watching.
Each woman looking at him
From the screen.
"Don't you hear my scream?"
"My shriek, even if I can't speak?"
"This is not my choice."
"This is not my voice."

What if you knew?
Would each moment
Have been different?

Did you know?
When you
Looked
And stared?

Do you know?
Each woman is scared.

Who else knows?
Fess up.
And let it go.
Let them go.
Help them get let go.

MultiMedia Collection
For A Digital Exposé

Accompanying Photograph
https://tinyurl.com/digitalexpose

PART SIX

Midnight

Daily we experience
So many blessings
We do not deserve,
But we remember
That God paid for our worth.

Because He died we can live.
And so as we care for each other,
Kindness we can give.

Don't ever be afraid
To lend a hand.
Don't be afraid to take a stand,
For the single, the widowed,
The orphaned, or the lame;
The blind, the weak,
Persecuted,
We are all the same.

The thing is
We are also the same
As the trafficked, the trafficker,
And the buyer.
Above each one,
God sees us no higher.

In His eyes,
We are all loved the same.
No matter our level of shame.

No matter whether
We are the victims,
Victors, oppressed,
Or oppressors,
The persecuted, persecutors,
Rescued, or rescuers.

At the core, we share brokenness
And the potential for beauty,
Even in our ugliest moments
Rooted in our nativity,
Rising like a Phoenix
Is always a possibility.

It's true that the uglier we seem,
The less likely we feel
It is possible to be redeemed.

But there is one who redeems all.
He took it all, see his skin skald.

There is no wound too deep,
That He could not feel.

There is no bad deed so great,
For which He has not already paid.

His heart bleeds for the trafficked,
The trafficker, and the buyer;
He calls each to come up higher.

He calls each to trust Him
With their souls,
And He yearns to call them

His own.

He also calls you,
And me.
He wants us to truly see,
The way He sees you and me.

He wants us to experience His love,
And embrace His truth
That rests on us from above.

We can deny Him all we want,
It won't diminish His pursuit.

PART SEVEN

Not My Brother

You speak
For me.
You manhandle
Me.
You tell the health care team
You are my brother.

You tell them a story
They are satisfied to believe.
One that you
Made up about me.
So many inconsistencies
They do not see.

If I am schizophrenic
And suicidal
And cut myself
At the wrists,
Why do my wrists
Look more like rope burns
Than healed knife wounds?

If I lock myself away
In my room
Always,
How did I
Become pregnant?

If you are always
With me,
How can you

Not know
Who the father is—
Of my baby
That I didn't get to have?

Since you tried to
Perform my abortion
Yourself
At your house—
My prison,
Why would you
Tell them
I am having
A miscarriage?

In any case,
They don't notice
The scars
Of different ages
On my torso,
Covered from public view—
Except when my
Private spaces
Become public,
With men
Brought in
By you.

After treating me
In the hospital
For a few days,
They have sent me
Back home
With you.

I can only
Think these thoughts.
I cannot
Write them—
My wrists are bound,
And I can hardly see.
It is dark in this small closet—
My prison cell.

Until one day
The police
Rescue me
When they raid
Your house
For drugs.

They didn't know
About me,
You see.
I was found
Peripherally.
They didn't know
I was
Your commodity.

Now I am free.

I wish every girl
Or boy
Or woman
Or man
Like me
Could see—
Trafficked

We don't have to be.
But once trapped in it,
No, we can't see.
The trafficker takes away
Our eyes,
You see—
Even our very identity.

We learn to love him,
You see,
And even defend
And protect him.

So you need to know
What to do
When you see me
And something seems fishy.

Follow your instinct.
Let me speak.
Suspect me.
Suspect him.
Let me speak—
With my mouth
And my body,
My scars
And my story.
Separate him
From me.
Find a way.
Find me.
Rescue me.
Save me.
Protect me.

Help me heal.
Be my healer.

PART EIGHT

Epilogue

We can deny it all we want,
This issue in our backyards
And on our front porch,
But now we know.

And now that we know,
What will we do?
Will we do something?

MULTIMEDIA LINKS

Thoughts On Human Trafficking

Video of Live Performance:
https://tinyurl.com/thoughtshumantrafficking

TEDx Pitch Night

Video of Live Performance:
https://tinyurl.com/tedxpitchnight

Audio Performance:
https://tinyurl.com/tedxpitchnightaudio

A Digital Exposé

Accompanying Photograph
https://tinyurl.com/digitalexpose

A Midnight Poem

Video of Live Performance:
https://tinyurl.com/amidnightpoem

OTHER MEDICAL HUMANITIES BOOKS

BY DR. SHERRY-ANN BROWN, DR. BROWN CARES LLC

The Healer Speaks: Poems For Patients, Students, Doctors, Nurses, Therapists, Educators, & Everyone Impacted By Medicine

Life & Death: Hope & Dignity

Just One More Step: Poems From Practicing Medicine & Science

D.R. B.R.A.V.E.: Poems From Medical Practice

Black Renaissance: Know Thyself, Heal The Land

& The Following Gift & Graduate Editions!

I Cannot Die Tonight: Medical Anthology
(Gift Composite Edition)
Includes: The Healer Speaks,
Life & Death: Hope & Dignity

I Cannot Die Tonight: Medical Anthology
(Graduate Edition For The Young Healer)
Includes: The Healer Speaks,
Life & Death: Hope & Dignity

Rise Now: Medical Anthology
(Gift Composite Edition)
Includes: D.R. B.R.A.V.E., Just One More Step

Rise Now: Medical Anthology
(Graduate Edition
For The Young Healer)
Includes: D.R. B.R.A.V.E., Just One More Step

Turn It On: Medical Anthology
(Gift Composite Edition)
Includes: The Healer Speaks, D.R. B.R.A.V.E.
Life & Death: Hope & Dignity

Turn It On: Medical Anthology
(Graduate Edition
For The Young Healer)
Includes: The Healer Speaks, D.R. B.R.A.V.E.
Life & Death: Hope & Dignity

CONNECT

Get Your **The Healer Speaks** Book Set
Tote And Other Gifts At

Www.LyricalMezzanine.Com/Shop

@LyricalMezz

DrBrownCares@Gmail.Com

@DrBrownCares

Www.DrBrownCares.Com

See testimonials at
Www.DrBrownCares.Com/Testimonials
&
Www.DrBrownCares.Com/Testimonials-2

Www.TinyUrl.Com/LyricalMezz
Www.TinyUrl.Com/CreativityMedicine

NOTES

www.ingramcontent.com/pod-product-compliance
Lightning Source LLC
Chambersburg PA
CBHW031502210526
45463CB00003B/1035

* 9 7 8 1 6 5 3 3 7 1 7 1 6 *